D1561364

# ARE YOU A GYM MOUSE?

Get Over Your Fears of the
Gym, Take Charge of
Your Lifestyle and
Become a More
Confident, Healthier You

Agi Kadar

The author can be contacted at
www.healthbalanced.com or
agi@healthbalanced.com

Cover design and formatting
by Diane Stimson
www.DianeStimson.com

# DISCLAIMER

This book is not intended as a substitute for the medical advice of physicians. The reader should regularly consult a physician regarding his or her health. Always check with your doctor before beginning this or any exercise, nutrition, or supplement program.

The opinions and statements made in this book are intended for informational use only. They are the author's opinions and are based on her experience. The information in this book is meant to educate and serve as an aid to the reader's health and well-being. They should not be considered as medical advice, diagnoses, or treatment.

The author and publisher of this material do not accept any liability or responsibility for any injury or damage that may occur through following the material and instructions in this book.

The activities described in this book may be too strenuous or dangerous for some people and the reader should consult a physician before engaging in them.

# DEDICATION

My husband Tibor, for all his love,
patience, and support.

My children, Andrea and Andrew
for believing in me.

# TABLE OF CONTENTS:

# ACKNOWLEDGEMENTS

There were so many people who inspired me to start writing. Thanks for all your support for making this book happen!

Carl, Shari, John, Anne and Stanley, Diane, Maya, Betsy, and all my friends and clients.

Thank you to the Self-Publishing School, and Chandler Bolt and Jaime Grodberg for giving me their support.
(https://xe172.isrefer.com/go/curcust/gymmouse07)

My Buddy, Sharon, for being only a phone call away.

Brianna for always listening and encouraging.

Thank you to my editors, Wayne Purdin, Stanley Boorman and Betsy Epstein for all their help.

Contact Agi at agi@healthbalanced.com or visit her website at www.healthbalanced.com

# INTRODUCTION:

Gym Mouse: Not a Gym Rat.
A Gym Mouse is a very capable person, who wants to work out and get in shape, but who is confused and not sure what to do in the gym. When a Gym Mouse joins a gym, he or she tends to hide on the treadmill or on the elliptical machine and not do much else. The Gym Mouse gets easily discouraged and disappointed by the lack of results and leaves the fitness center.

I have been in the fitness industry over 20 years and worked in the same gym for the last 16. I always had a heart for the Gym Mouse, the members who were scared and confused and just wanted to be healthy. I'm very happy to say that I helped a lot of them get started, stick with it, and even begin to like regular exercise.

Are you a Gym Mouse?

You know you need to exercise. Your doctor told you. Your family and friends told you. You have all the excuses in the world why you don't have the time, the money, the knowledge, the personality, and, most of all, the body to do it. Deep down, you know they're all excuses to justify that you're scared and intimidated. It's time to admit that you're not a gym rat; you're a Gym Mouse. It's okay. We can work with that.

Dear Gym Mouse,
The purpose of this book to reach more of you out there and help you get into a fitness routine. Please read my book with an open mind and give regular physical activity a chance! *Your life depends on it!* You have the power to improve your health and longevity by making choices that support a healthier lifestyle. Overcoming your fears now is easier than overcoming illness later. If you already have an illness, let's overcome both and make your life better!

It's time to decide for whom you're doing this? The Gym Rat, who intimidates you? Your co-worker who makes fun of you for making an effort? Or yourself, your health, your life, and your loved ones?

It's okay to be a gym mouse. You can still overcome your fears and start a healthy lifestyle that includes regular exercise in the gym. You don't have to become a gym rat to get stronger and healthier and have fun in the gym.

Unless you're a very motivated and disciplined person who also understands some basic fitness, you're better off joining a gym or health club than trying to do it yourself at home. Face it; you'll never stick with it.

Let me show you the smart way to do it! In this book, I'll show you how to find the best fitness facility for your needs and personality. I'll also show you how to defeat all your fears and excuses as to why you think you can't do this and how to turn them into motivation and fun.

I'll walk you through the sign up process so you'll know what to expect and get exactly the membership you need, no more, no less. I'll give you all the information so you can look forward to going to the gym and getting the most out of your membership and reaching your goals. I'll give you all the tips to help you enjoy going to the gym regularly and having a great relationship with staff and other members.

In my 16 years working in the same gym as a personal trainer and manager, I have seen hundreds of people come through the door looking for solutions but too scared to follow through and do the work.

I helped a lot of them to control, reverse, or prevent health problems and get in the best shape of their lives. As a lifestyle coach, I showed them how to change their habits and become the healthiest and fittest Gym Mouse they could be.

This book will show you that, aside from all the health benefits, exercising can be fun, and you'll be looking forward to your time spent in the club. You'll have more confidence, strength, endurance, and energy to do all the things you want to do and didn't think possible.

You don't need to have fitness or athletic dreams to start an exercise program. Just wanting to be healthier, be stronger, function better every day, and get more pleasure out of your life is a good enough goal. I'll help you find your dream, so you can find the motivation to do it.

My client, Jennifer, said I changed her life by helping her start an exercise program that helped her stop smoking. She used the money she would have spent on cigarettes for personal training. She gave up a dangerous habit for a healthy one.

I promise that after reading my book, you'll be able to pick the best facility for you and make the most of your membership. You'll be looking forward to your exercise time, feel better about yourself, and see your goals realized.

So don't wait! Start reading and start putting my tips to work for you. Imagine where you can be in a few weeks and months!

Read the book and change your life! The quicker you read it, the quicker you'll see results, feel the benefits, and become a healthier, stronger, and more confident Gym Mouse!

"The miracle isn't that I finished. The miracle is that I had the courage to start."
(John "the Penguin" Bingham)

Let's get started!

Chapter 1:
JOINING A GYM THE SMART WAY – TIPS
FROM AN INSIDER

So you're a Gym Mouse. It's alright. Not everybody is a Gym Rat or wants to become one. There are a lot of people like you out there. But you can still follow an exercise program and have a healthier, fitter body.

Your best bet is to join a gym where you can find expert help and support and meet others like you who will help you keep motivated.

Don't think you're alone. Most people are a little hesitant when they first join a gym. You feel like you expose yourself and your shortcomings to others if you're not an athlete. It's okay. Most people are just like you, just trying to get in shape or become healthier. The small percentage who are in great shape and know what they're doing are too busy doing it to judge you or care about what you're doing. Even if you feel like everyone is watching you, believe me, they're not. They're probably worrying about you watching and judging them. So relax and be proud of yourself for being there and working for your future. Be a proud Gym Mouse!

The first step is to find the right facility for you:

Check out what's available in your immediate area. It's very unlikely that you'll have to drive a great distance to workout every day.

With all the low-priced competition around, most gyms and health clubs have lowered their enrollment fees as well as their monthly dues. So, a membership is very reasonable and affordable. Of course, if you desire more luxuries, you can still find a high-end club where, for a substantial monthly fee, you can expect more services and amenities catering to your convenience.

Think about what you need to make you happy and to keep you coming back. Do you desire a good deal or more luxuries to keep you comfortable? Keep in mind that healthcare is much more expensive later when you spend a lifetime without taking care of your body.

A regular health club should provide enough for your basic needs with more amenities for an extra charge. So, you need to decide if your first concern is your budget or if you also want some pampering in the club. If your budget is your main concern, you need to first look into some of the chains with franchises and corporate gyms. There are some facilities that offer all the basics for a very affordable monthly fee.

If money isn't a concern and you want all the extras, look into some of the high-end clubs that have extra services and amenities included in their monthly dues. Shop around; check out all the facilities in your area. That way, you'll feel more comfortable when you're ready to make a decision.

What kind of environment do you find the most motivating and comfortable? Do you want a pool, tennis courts, racquetball, or basketball?

Individually owned franchises or private gyms might have more of a family atmosphere. They're more likely to have staff who have worked there for years and who get to know the members more. They're also more likely to go out of their way to make their members feel comfortable and happy.

Corporate gyms are likely to be more business oriented and bigger with a lot of members. That's not necessarily bad, but less intimate. But they might also offer more services than a smaller gym and you can also get membership options to use only one club or all of their other locations.

Managers are more pressured to meet the bottom line. They might be more aggressive and try to get you to buy personal trainings or other services.

There are also more specific, boutique gyms or studios that are offering fewer but more specific training options. Small personal training studios are great for the constant guidance of a trainer and have a smaller facility with no crowds, if that appeals to you and you have the resources to pay for it.

If you're new to exercise, you're probably better off with a conventional health club where you can try different things and have more variety. But if you're only interested in a certain form of exercise like yoga, Pilates, martial arts, cycling, or one-on-one personal training in a smaller setting, then you should find a studio just for that.

When you're looking for the right club for you, find out everything you can. Shop around so you can decide what's the best fit for you. Make some calls and ask questions about membership policies and fees. You can also get a feel on the phone to see if they care about you or are just pushing sales. I would still go and check to see in person if the information you get appeals to you. One salesperson won't represent the whole gym.

Make an appointment to meet with a fitness consultant. Let them go through their pitch and then ask questions. Find out about enrollment and any other sign-up or administrative fees. Ask if there are any different monthly fees or memberships.

Do they participate in any health insurance reimbursement programs or other programs offered for seniors where health insurance pays for their membership? Also, call your insurance company to find out what gyms they're participating with. You might be able to get some or all of your money back. Ask what they need from you or your gym. Some insurance companies want a printout from your club to prove how many times a month you go and how much you pay. They might have a required monthly visit you need to keep. Your employer might also offer a reimbursement program for health club memberships.

Find out about the cancellation policy: if there is any cancellation fee, how far in advance you have to cancel, and if it has to be in writing. Ask if there is a contract or some type of commitment, or you can cancel anytime. Some gyms sell a membership along with personal training. The membership may be cancelled but the personal training is a contract for one year with a higher monthly fee. Canceling your gym membership doesn't automatically cancel the contract.

Is there a yearly fee and when do they charge that? Some places make you pay that at the sign-up, so you have to put up a larger amount to get started. Some facilities have 1 or 2 designated months when they charge the yearly fee for everybody. Ask what is included in the membership and what else is offered such as childcare, unlimited towel service, or tanning. You might get a better deal on those if you add them to your membership at the sign up.

Also, ask about free introductory training sessions or orientation and introductory personal training packages. They might offer a special price for that only at the sign up. You are likely to get a good deal. How much is personal training after the intro? Are all personal trainers certified? Do you have a choice of a trainer for your orientation or will they assign one to you?

Ask about any additional programs for children, sports conditioning, or any other interest you or your family might have. Check the class schedule and childcare hours to make sure they suit your needs.

Ask about "freezes" (suspending your membership for medical or personal reasons). Do they have senior freezes for those who go south for the winter or north for the summer? Not all gyms offer a policy to freeze memberships for any kind of absence.

What is their guest policy? Can you bring your children to workout with you at a designated time, and what is the age limit for that?

Can you use other clubs in the same chain? You might need a travel pass to do that. Is there an extra charge for that? Do they have a timeframe to get your money back if you're not satisfied? Some places give you 10-14 days for that from the time of your sign up.

Before you make your decision, ask for a

free pass for a week or at least for a day so you can experience the atmosphere and get a closer look at the employees and the members. Talk to people. Take a class if you can; find out about the instructors' and trainers' qualifications. Try to go at the time of day you would regularly go so you can see how crowded the workout floor is and see the ages of the clientele at that time.

Make sure you have a doctor's clearance to start exercising, especially if you have any medical conditions, have been sedentary for a long time, have any recent injuries or physical limitations, or are over 65 years old. The doctor might give you some guidelines to follow to safely start an exercise program.

You'll have to answer medical questions when you sign up. If you have or had certain conditions, the club might require you to bring a note from your doctor that you're cleared to work out. You can bring that right away so you can save time and get started.

Share any limitations or problems you have so they can help you with a safer and better program when you start your training.

When you feel satisfied, sign up! Read everything before signing. Make sure what's written down is the same as what you agreed on verbally with the fitness consultant. Get a copy of everything for your records.

Congratulations! You made a life changing decision! Now let's make the best of it!

I bet you didn't know there are many ways to get your money's worth, and even end up saving money by joining your local health club.

Let's say they offer free coffee. You have 2 or 3 cups every day, and you never have to pay for coffee again. You can most likely drink your membership fee in coffee every month.

Some gyms have a little basket of mints at the front desk. Take a handful every day and, by Halloween, you'll have enough candy for your trick-or-treaters.

If you take a shower there every day, you can add to your savings by not using your hot water at home, drying your hair with the hair dryer in the locker room, and not having to buy soap or shampoo ever again. You can even sell your hairdryer and coffee machine at a yard sale.

I think by now you can see how smart it is to join a gym. It's affordable and a very reasonable thing to do. You'll have access to equipment and expert help and meet people just like you. It will be a fun and rewarding experience.

So let's get to the best part! Let's see the best way to get started!

Chapter 2:
CONGRATULATIONS! YOU JOINED THE
CLUB. NOW WHAT?

Be proud of yourself for taking this important, possibly life-changing step. You've made the first step toward a healthier and happier life. Now, you might as well make the best of it.

You're doing something for yourself, for your health, and for your future. Look at it as an investment in your health and your body. You only get one body, no returns, no exchanges. You're responsible to take care of it so it lasts for a long life. Your body is the reflection of your lifestyle!

It doesn't matter how slow you go; you're still going faster than people sitting on the couch!

It's okay to be a Gym Mouse. It's okay if you're not crazy about exercise. That's why you're here. You're not alone. As it might look intimidating at the beginning, the best place for you to be is in an environment with people to help you, guide you, and keep you motivated. I'm confident that if you can stick with it for a while, you might even find it fun.

So let's see what you need to get started!

Make sure you eat a snack before you go if it's first thing in the morning or if it has been a long time since your last meal. You don't want to be too full but want some fuel in your tank. Experiment with different foods before exercise. Some people can tolerate more food than others before physical activity. Find what works best for you.

You will need to drink water before, during and after your workout. Bring a water bottle with you to the gym and take small sips while exercising. Coconut water is a great natural way to add carbohydrates for energy and to replenish electrolytes lost through sweating. The more you sweat, the more you will need to hydrate.

If you have medical considerations like diabetes or hypoglycemia, consult your doctor for proper nutrition guidelines for your workouts.

You should also have a snack after vigorous exercises, to replenish nutrients and energy stores. It's recommended to eat a protein- and carbohydrate-containing snack within 30 minutes of a workout. It's especially important if you were doing high-intensity intervals or strength training. If you were sweating, elevated your heart rate, and were breathing heavily during your workout, you'll need a recovery snack, like a protein shake or bar, to repair muscle damage. If you just did some light activity or went for a walk, your regular meal will suffice.

Next, you need to have the right attire. Athletic shoes are a must! They also should fit the occasion. Your 5-year-old tennis shoes you cut the grass in won't do! Come on; you're saving all that money. So, invest in some well-fitting, supportive sneakers.

Cross trainers are probably good for most occasions, but if you have special goals or needs, you need to get a specific type of footwear. The gym training staff can help with any questions you have.

If you want to mostly walk or run, you need walking or running shoes. If you're only interested in Zumba or dance classes, you need shoes for that. Regular fitness sneakers will stick to the floor when you twist your feet or try to pivot and they will hurt your knees and hips. (I'll go into more details on what you need for each class later.)

If you have special conditions, such as flat feet, high arches, supinating or pronating feet, injuries, or other medical problems, consult your doctor or an expert on footwear. You don't want to be sidelined right away because of injury from inappropriate shoes. If you wear orthotics or custom-made shoe inserts, you most likely need to wear them for exercise. Make sure they fit your fitness shoes. Ask your doctor for advice if you're unsure.

Workout clothes are easier. They just need to be comfortable and appropriate for the exercise. If it motivates you to wear nice, matching new workout clothes, go for it! Do what it takes!

If you don't really care, any clean, comfortable, well-fitting sweats and T-shirts will do.

If you're usually hot and sweat a lot, it might be worth investing in a few sport shirts made of wicking materials. They help remove moisture from the shirt and keep you cool and dry. In that case (the case of sweating buckets—which is, by the way, a good thing most of the time) you also want to make sure to rub a little extra detergent where the shirts come in contact with your armpits, when you launder them. That material likes to hold onto body odor after a while.

Personal hygiene rules apply. Wear deodorant, but don't use strong fragrances when you work out. Others might be sensitive or allergic and when they're breathing harder, they just want clean air.

It's a good idea to have a couple of layers until you figure out what the temperature in your health club is and how long it takes you to warm up. You don't want to be too hot, but if you get cold easily, it's good to have a sweatshirt handy in case the air conditioning is too cold for you or you end up near a fan.

Bring a water bottle with you or some cash to buy water. You should stay well hydrated while working out. If the facility has a water fountain, then you can use that too.

A small workout towel can be handy to wipe your face or moisten and wrap around your neck to keep cool.

There are other accessories you can get now or later as you see the need: gloves, wraps, and supports for knees, wrists, etc. for old or recent injuries if they're warranted.

Ask someone to show you the locker room and the available amenities in there. If you're using a locker, you might need a lock, or you can leave your valuables at home or in the car. There are some easier combination locks with numbers that line up instead of having to turn them in different directions. If you still have trouble, ask front desk personnel if they can add your combination to your account info in case you cannot open your lock.

If you're taking a shower at the gym, know what they offer and what you need to bring from home for your routine. Most places have at least soap, shampoo, and hairdryers. High-end clubs usually give you even more hygiene products and towels. Check before you pack your gym bag.

Next, make an appointment with one of the trainers for your first orientation. Show up on time for the appointment. Call if you're late or cannot make it as soon as you know. Respect the time of the trainer.

Ask a staff member or the personal trainer at your appointment to show you around so you can get to know where everything is in your club.

There should be an area for cardio equipment. It might be called the cardio deck if it's on a raised platform.

Most of the cardio machines now have

televisions attached to them, so you can watch your favorite program while you're working out. You'll need headphones to listen, or you can use closed captioning if available.

They should also have an iPod dock so you can listen to your own music. Ask the staff if you need a password to access wifi if you want to listen to online music.

Some gyms have a cardio-theater where they will play movies in a somewhat dark room. You can watch a film while you're walking on the treadmill or biking.

There should be a circuit training area where the weight machines are lined up. This is what they will most likely show you at your orientation.

There should be a free weight area or room, where the dumbbell and barbell racks and benches should be. There also may be a squat rack, Smith machine, or plate-loaded machines. The trainer can show you what they are, but you'll need proper instructions and practice when you decide to use them later on.

Bigger clubs might have an area designated only for female exercises.

There should be one or more aerobic rooms or studios where the classes are held. There might be a separate bike room for cycle classes and a yoga or Pilates studio. Ask if you can use the rooms when there are no classes going on. So, if you need some quiet time, you can go in there to stretch or do some floor exercises.

The trainer should sit down with you and ask you to fill out a form about your health and fitness history. They should, at least, talk to you about it and ask you questions. They need to know what your current conditioning or de-conditioning is, to design a personalized fitness program. Make sure to mention any injuries, discomforts, pain, or physical limitations, and medications that can alter your heart rate or influence your exercise intensity in any way. Also, tell them if you have any special instructions from your doctor or physical therapist.

They should ask you if you want to take your measurements and body fat percentage to keep on file so you can see your progress. The trainer also should perform a fitness and flexibility test to assess your fitness level.

During the session, ask questions and make sure you understand the exercises they're teaching you. Ask them to write down seat and machine settings and any other notes or clues, so that you can remember and do the training properly on your own.

They should show you some of the cardio equipment that will suit you best to get started, and should show you how to warm up. Then they should introduce you to some of the circuit machines to start building your strength. Ask them to include exercises that benefit you in your everyday life and functioning.

Your starter program should be an overall body-conditioning program that includes all the major muscle groups, but won't take you longer than 30-45 minutes to complete, including some cardio. Avoid overdoing it in the beginning, and gradually increase your intensity and time spent working out. You should be comfortable with everything they show you.

After your session, make an appointment for the second training in 1-3 weeks. Don't wait too long but give yourself a little time to familiarize yourself with the program before you try to learn more if you plan on doing it on your own. Keep track of your workouts to record your progress.

When you take your second orientation with the personal trainer, ask their advice on how to safely increase intensity in your program so that you'll keep seeing results. By now, you should have an idea what's a reasonable time you can spend at the gym and how often you'll make it there. Knowing your schedule will make it easier to plan a program.

Set reasonable weekly goals, even if it's just showing up and walking for 15 minutes in the first few weeks. You're forming a new habit, and making permanent changes takes time. It's supposed to take 21 days to make a habit or break a habit. So make a contract with yourself that you'll go to the gym for at least 21 days to build that habit. If you can do it for 21 days, then you can definitely keep going after that.

If you can budget it, I highly recommend that you buy some personal training sessions. It will keep you more accountable, more motivated, and right on track toward your results. When a personal trainer shows you what to do and takes you into that dreaded free weight area, you'll realize it's not so bad. It's very doable and even more fun than just using the machines. It will also build your confidence when you see how much you're capable of.

I'll talk about how to pick your personal trainer and your training schedule in a later chapter.

Consider what the best time is for you to visit the health club. There are usually slightly different age groups at different times of the day. Unless you're forced to go at a certain time, choose the time when you feel most comfortable or it is most convenient for you to go. You want to have most of the circumstances in your favor, so that you're encouraged to go and can build a habit of a healthy and active lifestyle.

Usually, early mornings are more business-like. People need to get to work so they want to get their workout done. There isn't as much socializing and wasting time. But you'll see the same friendly faces every day and get to know the people.

A little later, the retired crowd will start to trickle in. They workout, socialize a bit, have coffee together, and have their little country club. It could be a nice way to make some new friends, workout, and socialize at the same place. Friends will keep you more accountable and motivated to keep going to the gym.

After school starts, parents will be coming in and dropping off little ones at the daycare. This time will get a bit busier, because classes will be starting too.

Then, by noon, the place will quiet down a little bit.

If you have a long lunch time and you work close to the club, you might want to try that time if it works for you. The place most likely won't be crowded. Just figure in your shower time.

After high school is dismissed, you'll see more students in the weight room. That might be the time to avoid if you don't like loud laughing and talking teenagers around you.

Then there might be a short lull before the evening rush starts. Most places are the busiest at night after work, but it can still be a great experience. Some people like the energy and faster pace of the nighttime. You'll meet all kinds of people, there are probably more classes to choose from than in the morning, and you can learn how to share equipment with others and play nice.

Before closing, there will be less people working out again. If you're a night owl and don't go to bed early, this might be the perfect time. Regular exercise will help you get a better night's sleep, regardless of what time of day you work out, by reducing stress and anxiety. For most people, exercising in the evening won't cause any problems with falling asleep, but it's more important to keep a regular bedtime schedule that your body is used to. But if you're one of those individuals who gets so energized after vigorous exercise, that it takes a while to wind down, plan to have 2-3 hours of quiet time before bed. Test out all available options and see what works best for you and your lifestyle, regardless of what the clock says. If you're suffering from insomnia, talk to your doctor about the best possible time for exercise to work with your treatment.

So now you know the basics of how to get started. It's getting more exciting and interesting as you learn more about this new adventure. The more you know the less scary it will be.

Let's keep going on this exciting journey to a fitter, healthier, and braver Gym Mouse and see how to pick a personal trainer, who can make this experience even more fun and rewarding for you.

Chapter 3:
CHOOSING A PERSONAL TRAINER

After you do your orientation or circuit trainings, it's time to decide if you can invest in some personal training. I highly recommend it, unless you have the experience, knowledge and motivation to do it on your own.

In a perfect world, everyone would have a personal trainer at least 3 times a week. I know it's not always possible. But if we want something badly enough, we can make it happen.

Since I have been a personal trainer, I hear every week how much difference a personal trainer can make in a person's life. Besides motivating you, keeping you safer, and making the gym time more enjoyable and fun, the trainer will keep you more accountable and more likely to stick to your routine. They will help you set reasonable and obtainable goals and make you work harder to help you reach your results faster. Even clients who are very motivated, and work out on their own, tell me all the time that they workout harder under the watchful eyes of a personal trainer.

If it's not in your budget, see what you can do to afford it:
> * Ask your family and friends for gift certificates for personal trainings for all occasions when they would give you presents.
> * Stop smoking and use the money for training.
> * Give up soda or junk food to save up the money.
> * Cut back on eating out or going out to save some money.
> * Make your coffee in the morning to take it on the road instead of stopping at the coffee shop.
> * Have a yard sale or take some items to a consignment shop.

If you liked the trainer you did the orientations with, go ahead and schedule your sessions. If you're not sure or didn't feel comfortable, find another trainer. You can also switch at any time, even after starting your trainings.

Ask the front desk staff or the fitness consultants for their opinion. They might recommend someone who would be a better fit for you. Ask other members who do training sessions and have been coming to this gym for a while.

Watch how the personal trainers work with their clients. Ask them questions when they're free. Ask if they can give you 5-10 minutes to show you an exercise, and see if you "click."

Talk to several trainers. Find out about their certifications and anything they specialize in. Ask them questions to see what they're passionate about. Get a feel for their personalities to see if they're a match for yours.

You want to feel comfortable with your instructor, you want to trust them and feel confident that they're there for you and they want the best for you. You'll spend a lot of time with them. You'll expose your weaknesses and fears to them.

Can they make you forget how self-conscious you are? Can they make you relax and enjoy the session? Can they motivate you to work hard? Do you trust them and their instructions? Do you like them enough to spend time with them over and over again?

There are a lot of personal trainers who genuinely care for their client's well-being and progress. Don't give up if you don't click with the first trainer. Just as you don't become best friends with every person you meet, you might have to put in a little time and effort to find the best fitness professional for you. But when you find them, it could be a life-changing experience.

It's important that they ask you questions to learn your health and fitness history. Even though they should have your information from your orientation, they should go over any special considerations, health concerns, or injuries with you.

They should also ask you about your goals and dreams and tell you about how they plan to help you achieve them. They should discuss a plan with you, how often you need to see them, and what you need to do to see the results you're looking for. You should reassess the plan from time to time.

If you cannot train regularly, ask their opinion of a strategy you can implement to make it work. Maybe you can do 3 to 6 trainings in the first 2 or 3 weeks to start with, then spread them out a bit and see how you do on your own for 1 or 2 weeks, and then meet again to get advice on how to proceed.

Once you have a base conditioning and have learned to do certain exercises correctly, you can spread your sessions to once a week or even every other week, just to keep you on track and going forward. As long as you can keep yourself motivated, it could be a very successful program. But if at any time, you feel yourself slipping off the wagon, you should seek out your personal trainer's help to get back on schedule. It's much easier to keep going than to start over again. Also, don't waste the time and money you've already invested in your fitness to stop and have to do it over again.

Ask about bigger packages for a better price. Most places will give you a discount if you buy "in bulk." Usually, you have a year to use up the sessions after purchase, but find out your gym's policy, so you don't lose them.

I would recommend starting with a few one-hour sessions that would include some cardio training and plenty of time to get a good workout while making sure you learn the proper form for lifting and stretching at the end. Once you get some conditioning, you can switch to 30-minute trainings, step up the intensity, and cut back on time.

Another way to save money is to do partner or group training.
Find out if they offer small group personal training. If they don't, you can always suggest it or talk to other members and see if they would be interested. Then approach a trainer or a manager with the idea. Or find

just one more person who wants to do training and would like to partner with you. With a partner or a group, you can save money, have fun with others, and make friends who can motivate you and keep you even more accountable.

I have been doing group trainings for years and I see my clients enjoy the spirit of friendship while they work out together for similar goals and they are happy for each other's gains. Strength in numbers makes them more comfortable and less intimidated while trying new things and helps them believe they can do it. It also makes them want to show up, because they know others are counting on them.

Be courteous and respectful of your trainer's time and money. Understand that this is their main income. If they don't train, they usually don't get paid, or they earn very low wages. Give them enough time if you need to cancel your session, so they can schedule someone else. Cancel last minute only for emergencies or illness.

Find out the cancellation policy. Some places will charge you all or a partial amount of the training price if you cancel less than 24 hours before the appointment. Some owners leave it to the discretion of the trainer. If you cancel "just because," tell them to charge you. This is their livelihood. Just imagine you go to work, ready for a presentation, and at the last minute, they tell you that you don't need to do it but you won't get paid for it either, but hang around because, in an hour, you'll need to work again on something else.

A good personal trainer also does his or her "homework" and gets ready for the training in advance. So, they have already put some time and work into it before you even show up. Don't leave them hanging.

I usually try to work with my clients. I understand that things happen that are out of their control. If it only happens occasionally and is for a good reason, I don't charge them. Also, some try to make up the session, on another day or another time. If you do your part, the trainer will be more understanding of your circumstances.

It's a great idea to have a personal trainer and they can greatly enhance your gym experience and your motivation. You'll be looking forward to your training sessions with them and see a lot better and quicker results.

Next, we will go over some gym etiquette and rules to make you feel comfortable and at home at your club and fit in with the members and staff even more.

Chapter 4:
GYM ETIQUETTE - THE WRITTEN AND
THE UNWRITTEN RULES

There are certain "rules" you need to be aware of when working out at a health club. Following them will make your experience much better, and you'll be more respected and liked by staff and other members alike. Some might be obvious and common sense; some you might not think of, if you have never belonged to a similar facility before. I think that most of them will be obvious once you think about them. I will spell them out anyway so that you can look like an experienced Gym Mouse.

Be courteous and respect other people's space, time, and workouts. Say hello, but don't hold them up by socializing. Most people are there to workout only. If you want to talk and see or make friends, do it at the juice bar or the locker room. Don't interrupt someone's workout. That's also true for staff and trainers. If they're working out, they're off the clock, and deserve peace as much as you do. If you have questions, find staff who are working. They will love you and respect you for the consideration you show them.

Wait for the trainers to finish working with their clients, before you talk to them or find one who is available if you need help, or ask someone at the desk. If it's your personal trainer you need to communicate with, leave them a message or talk to them when they're free.

Wear clean and neat workout clothes. Wearing street clothes or jeans with zippers can rip the upholstery on the equipment or get caught on something.  Wear appropriate footwear. Boots, sandals, or flip-flops can be dangerous and can get you injured. Also, wearing too much jewelry can hurt you. Rings can cause blisters and chains can get caught on machines or weights.

Practice good hygiene, use a deodorant but no heavy perfumes or cologne.

Bring a towel to keep you from dripping sweat all over. Use the paper towels and spray bottles to disinfect machines and equipment after use. They should be found at a few easily accessible places throughout the workout floor.

Don't litter. There should be plenty of trash cans for paper towels, tissues, or snack wrappers. Don't leave them around. Recycle your used bottles.

Share the equipment and weights. Working with other members is expected when the gym is busy. Ask before you jump in.

Don't just sit on machines if you see others waiting; don't text or read and hold up equipment. Using a cell phone for calls on the workout floor can be very distracting. Move to the juice bar, hallway, or locker room if you need to make a call.

Leave your phone in the locker when you take a class. Besides respecting the instructors and other members, give yourself some time off from the outside world. You deserve some uninterrupted time for yourself.

If you're listening to your own music, make sure you're not singing out loud. You might be a good singer, but this isn't a karaoke bar.

You shouldn't loudly grunt, moan, belch, etc.

Don't throw plates and weights. Don't slam them. Clean up after yourself; put them back on the racks when you're done. Wipe off mats and benches after using them. Leave them the way you like to find them yourself.

When taking a class, respect the space of the other participants. Leave enough room so you don't hit or knock into others during the workout.

Get to the class on time and stay until the end. Follow instructions. Don't bring bags, jackets, boots, or anything else you won't use in the class. Putting them on the classroom floor can make you or others trip or fall. Leave them in the locker room or cubbies, if available.

Practice common sense clean up in the locker room. Don't leave your things all over, especially sweaty clothes. Leave room for others on the bench and the counter. Share the mirrors and hairdryers. Rinse the shower and wipe the sink after yourself. You would not want to find them messy either. Let staff know if supplies are needed.

If you're not sure of some of the policies or rules, ask the staff or long-time members. They will be happy to help you.

Common sense and common courtesy go a long way. Just ask yourself: "What would I do if this were my home, and how would I like to be treated?" If you can keep to that, you'll be the most popular Gym Mouse in that facility.

Now that you can play by the rules, let's get started and see how much fun exercising can be if you make the gym your playground.

Chapter 5:
DO IT NOW!  HAVE FUN!  MAKE THE GYM
YOUR PLAYGROUND!

Don't wait! There will never be a better time
to start than right now. You'll always be
busy; life is always going to be there with
challenges and excuses. You can decide to
overcome those and make yourself and your
health a priority. By investing this time and
effort to become healthier and fitter, you'll be
able to give more to your family, your job,
and any other area that requires your
attention. So make the time to do it, make it
fun, and stick with it!

Don't let anyone steal your wind! They just
want to justify their own excuses, so don't let
them pull you down. Instead, challenge them
to join you. You might find the best workout
partner that way.

Don't be intimidated by people who are fit
and know what they're doing. They had to
start one day, just like you. Practice gives
confidence. You'll get there too. It doesn't

mean you need to become a gym rat. You'll be a confident, healthy Gym Mouse!

I'm sure you have overcome bigger things in your life, conquered much bigger fears than going to the gym. You can do this. What if there are people who look better, who are in better shape than you in the gym? That's okay. If they judge you, that's their problem. You should be proud of yourself for doing something that will benefit yourself, your health, and your future.

Even if this is your first time in a health club or it has been a long time since you belonged to a gym, it doesn't matter. You can do it! What do you have to lose? Let's see: weight, flabbiness, weakness, fear, self-consciousness just to name a few. Sounds like a good trade to me.

When you look around, you'll see that most of the intimidated exercisers are on the treadmill or the elliptical machines in their safe-zone, where they can hide under their headphones, behind the TV screen so they don't even have to talk to or see anyone or be seen by anyone. For them, it will get old and boring very soon, with no real results after a while. They will be still doing the same thing in a couple years -- if they don't quit -- and they will look and feel the same way. I've seen it often. Don't let that happen to you! You're here to have fun while improving your health and lifestyle. You're already here, might as well step out of your comfort zone and do it well.

Try different things.

You should have a beginner's workout from your orientation session with a personal trainer. Try it out as soon as you can after the training session while it's still fresh in your mind. Check the workout card and work through the circuit. Check seat and machine settings. Read the instructions on the machines. Look at the pictures; learn what muscle groups you're supposed to use. Make sure that's where you feel the exercise. If you're in doubt, ask a trainer or staff member on duty. It's much easier to learn the right way the first time, than try to fix bad habits later or, even worse, getting hurt. It's much more embarrassing to wait for an ambulance because you got hurt from your own neglect, than to ask for help.

Everybody started from the beginning at some point. That's why you joined the gym, so you have access to expert help.

I highly recommend that you get a few sessions with a certified personal trainer to make you more comfortable and safe doing your workouts.

Find an exercise buddy. Maybe someone you see in the gym at the same time. See if they want to partner up to meet at the gym and keep each other accountable. Just make sure you don't end up talking more than working out. You're here to motivate each other and maybe feel more comfortable on the workout floor or to try a new class together, drawing strength in numbers.

Get to know the staff, the trainers, and instructors. They'll also motivate you to come, "scold" you if you don't show up for a while, and help you to stay on track. After a while, you'll feel you don't want to let them down by not coming.

Look for other motivating club activities. Participate in challenges and events. Sometimes, they're for a good cause; sometimes, it's just to motivate members. Sign up for everything you can, just keep moving along.

Try different cardio machines. It will make your workout more exciting and you'll get more results by providing a variety of exercises for your body. It will also help you to avoid a plateau or overuse injuries, and keep you motivated.

Participate in different classes. Try everything at least once. Maybe try different instructors if the first one just didn't click for you. Give the classes a chance. They can be very motivating and lots of fun. Time will fly by and you'll make some new friends for sure.

You can also combine classes and the circuit. If you're taking a cycle class, which will be harder on your lower body, use some upper body machines for 15 minutes before or after the class. This way you get a more rounded workout.

If you're taking a strength or sculpting class, do 15-20 minutes cardio before. It will thoroughly warm you up and you'll get more out of your time at the club.

You can also combine cardio and circuit workout. Warm up 5-10 minutes on one of the machines, then do one round on the circuit machines. Go back to cardio for 5-10 minutes, then back to the circuit again. Do 2 to 3 sets using a different cardio machine each time. Time will go by really fast and you'll get a great workout.

Keep an exercise journal or card, where you can track your workouts. It will show your progress, the change in the weights you lifted, repetitions and sets you did. It can also be quite motivating to see check marks and cards and pages filling up as you're working out consistently.

I personally get great satisfaction checking or crossing out my workouts for the day. Sometimes I make an index card with a square representing each of my daily workouts for the week or the month. Then, when I'm done, I highlight the box. I use different colors for the different activities, like cardio, strength, class, etc. It looks really cool when you have a month worth of colored boxes. You can color them for any physical activity. Bike ride with the kids, hiking with your spouse, walking with your friends, etc. Shoot for a colored box for every day. Don't break the streak. You can even do jumping jacks and push-ups and bodyweight squats in front of the TV if there's a must-watch game or show on and you didn't get a chance to work out that day. Nobody said you have to sit when you're watching your favorite program.

Try to get at least 30 minutes of activity every day and watch those colored boxes multiply. You can also use a calendar. Put it on the wall where you see it several times a day to remind you. Then, every month you don't break your streak, reward yourself with a new water bottle, weightlifting gloves, cool socks, a new workout shirt, a fitness tracker or a massage.

Don't overdo it. Make sure to include active rest days. Walking, playing ball outside with your kids, or taking the dog for a longer walk. Not every day has to be a formal workout in the health club, but staying active on your rest days will make it easier to return to the gym and your workout routine the next day. It will reinforce your new active lifestyle as a habit. Just keep in mind that reasonable exercise will help your stress management, but adding too much exercise to an already stressful lifestyle can make it worse. I'll talk about that in the next chapter.

Tell everyone you know that you joined the gym. Be proud of it. It will make you more accountable. The more people you tell the less likely you want to stop and admit failure to them. Do what you have to do to make yourself go. You won't regret it in the long run.

Challenge friends or family members, even if they live far away, and compare workouts and experiences in the gym. See who keeps meeting goals and reward each other with a cool gift. Maybe meet to go to a game every few months you both keep up your fitness commitment.

Sometimes, people who think they hate it in the beginning will become the most dedicated gym goers after a while. You won't know if you like it if you don't give it a fair chance. You know you can do it, so let's get to it!

In the next chapter, I'll talk about cardiovascular training, how important it is, how to do it smart, and how to make it interesting. You don't have to spend your life doing cardio and getting bored out of your mind. Read the next chapter to see how cardio workouts can be quick, exciting, and enjoyable.

Chapter 6:
THE BRIGHT SIDE OF CARDIOVASCULAR TRAINING

Most people think that to lose weight or to get in shape, you need to do a lot of cardiovascular exercise. Hours of it on the treadmill or on the elliptical and on the cross trainer machines with a low intensity. It's old school. It's a waste of time. It's boring. It's not necessary. We can make cardio workouts fun and quick.

I've heard it all over the years: "I'll just start with cardio exercise." "I'll do strength after I lose the weight." I'll try a class after I get in shape." Yes, you can lose weight with cardio exercises or with dieting alone, but you'll stay the same shape and flabby, just maybe slightly smaller with saggy skin. Why suffer doing endless cardio workouts when there's a better way? Why shouldn't you get in shape, lose weight, get stronger, and have fun doing a variety of workouts at the same time? Wouldn't you also want to get toned, add some muscle, and strengthen your bones also?

Wouldn't you like to spend less time doing cardio and see more results? You're in luck! That's exactly what you'll need to do. You won't have to spend hours upon hours working out. You just need to do it the right way. Cardio and strength training together.

Even the Centers for Disease Control recommends at least 2.5 hours a week of moderate intensity aerobic exercise but only 75 minutes of vigorous intensity aerobic exercise. So the harder you work the shorter the duration you need to do it!

First, we start with the cardio. It's usually easier for everyone to learn and it's less intimidating. Most people can easily walk on the treadmill or ride a stationary bike. Even the elliptical or the rowing machines don't require a degree to master them. It is okay to start with what you feel comfortable doing.

We have established in the beginning that you're a Gym Mouse, so my guess is you're not looking to train for an Olympic event just yet. We're here to get you in shape and in the best health and functioning possible for the demands of everyday life, so you can handle stress and challenges like a champion. But if you change your mind later and want more, there's no reason why you couldn't pursue higher athletic goals.

When you're under stress, your body switches to "flight or fight" mode. You heart rate will increase, your cortisol, the stress hormone, will rise to get you ready to run away from danger or face it head on and fight. In the gym, cardio interval training will be your flight and strength training will be your fight. They both have to be intense enough to get you ready for anything and to teach you to recover fast so you can get back to normal as soon as you're done.

You want to teach your body to be able to work hard for a period of time with high intensity and then to return to normal quickly. Long moderate cardio won't make you strong enough, and it will drain you, stress you out, and make you tired instead of energizing you. You need to do shorter, more intense intervals to train your body the right way. Too long a high-intensity workout, on the other hand, can also be stressful and exhausting. That's why intervals are the best: mixing high intensity with rest periods.

The only reason you need to spend hours doing cardio exercises is if you're training for a marathon or an ironman triathlon or some other endurance event. Otherwise, less will yield more results. If your goals are to get in shape, lose weight, and get stronger and more energetic, you'll need to do little bit of both, cardio and strength. There's no need to spend hours on either one if you do it right. You just need to work hard enough to challenge your body to adapt without exhausting it and injuring it, so it will be able to respond to the stress of everyday living.

There's a great way to do that: "Do until you can't and rest until you can." Start out with working as hard as you can as long as you can and then rest until you can do it again. Best way to start is on a stationary bike. You can quickly add and reduce resistance and increase and decrease speed as needed. Start out with 30 seconds to a minute at hard intensity and as long a recovery as you need to do it again. As you get stronger, you can decrease your rest time and still keep the intensity on the intervals. Make sure there's always a clear difference between the 2 types of interval intensities. You don't want to blur the lines or you will end up with a boring cardio workout.

If you're using the treadmill or a step-mill machine, find the interval program to quickly change intensities or it might take you too long between changes and you won't get the desired results. A rowing machine can be a great tool also. Because it is an overall body exercise, it will quickly raise the intensity and can be easily used for intervals.

You can do intervals with body-weight exercises such as jumping jacks, burpees, and jump roping. On days when you can't get to the gym, you can do those at home. Even 12-15 minutes will be great to energize you and keep you on track.

I'll give you some ideas at the end of the book to get started and more details on advanced workouts in my next book about easy-to-follow workout programs for the Gym Mouse.

Some classes are set up as intervals for the most part, like cycle class and boot camp. You can also modify any class to your purpose. More on that in the chapter covering classes.

Always think about intensity. You'll need to get out of your comfort zone a bit. You'll need to focus on what you want to make stronger. If it's your cardiovascular system, you need to challenge that; if it's your muscles, you need to work them harder. If you can already do an exercise easily, your body has no need to get stronger, no need to adapt; you can already do it. Our bodies adapt to challenges. If you're used to walking, bike or run. Use the incline to make the workout harder. Shorter time with more intensity or interval training is your answer.

You can use a heart rate monitor or your perceived exertion to gauge your intensity. Most cardio machines have a heart-rate sensor. You can use that from time to time to check your heart rate, but try not to hold onto it the whole time. There are also heart rate monitors with a chest strap that will also work with most cardio equipment. You can see your heart rate without holding onto the machine. And now, heart rate monitors and fitness trackers are available with only a "watch" that monitors your heart rate on your wrist. You can also set them to your target heart rate.

There are charts on all cardio machines and some gym walls that show a target heart rate for all age groups.

They're based on the following formula: 220 minus your age being your maximum heart rate. Recommended range for a healthy person is to work out between 60% and 80% of their maximum heart rate. (I'll talk about modifying that for special conditions and ages in a later chapter, including safety guidelines for pregnant exercisers,)

But even healthy people are different and have different resting heart rates, which will affect their maximum heart rate, regardless of age. Also, the better shape you get in, the better shape your heart will be in. It will be able to pump more blood with each heartbeat, lowering your resting heart rate. Discuss recommended heart rates for you with your doctor.

Most fitness trackers can be set to show your target heart rate and the heart rate zone you're exercising in. You can also go back later and see what you did. That can help you and your doctor and personal trainer to modify your future workouts.

Even if you're using your heart rate as a guide to intensity, you can also use the "talk test" to make it more accurate for you.

Moderate intensity: able to talk, but not sing. Vigorous intensity: only able to say single words without pausing to breathe.

There is also the Rate of Perceived Exertion (RPE) Scale.

On a scale of 1-10:

Level

10 - being out of breath, maximum effort
     (cannot talk)

9 - very hard (single word only)

8 - hard (short sentence)

7 - somewhat hard (longer sentence)

6 - moderate (short conversation)

5 - easy

4 - very easy

High or moderate impact cardio workouts will also strengthen your bones, due to the impact and pounding. Low impact exercises not so much. Long, moderate cardio exercise will drain your body and can weaken bones. Keep the workouts short, but intense. Listen to your body and always work out at the intensity you're capable of on that day. Some days, you'll be stronger than others. Don't get hung up on the numbers. Do what your body is telling you. Remember: "Work until you can't and rest until you can!"

Cardiovascular conditioning is necessary but should not be the only way you try to get in shape. Strength training is very important and excellent for bone strength and prevention of osteoporosis. It will add muscle to your frame and raise your metabolism to burn more calories even when resting. It's also the next step you need to learn to round out your program to tone and tighten your body to be a better-looking and healthier Gym Mouse.

Chapter 7:
STRENGTH TRAINING – NOT JUST FOR
THE GYM RAT

As I told you in the previous chapter, cardiovascular exercise is just not enough to get you or keep you in shape, even if that just looks safer and easier to do. You'll need to blend resistance training into your routine to get the most out of your exercise regimen and strengthen your muscles, bones, tendons, and ligaments.

It's okay to start with the cardio machines first when you get to the gym to warm up and prepare yourself for your workout. Think through what you're going to do and get your mind and body ready. Forget the outside world, and enjoy taking care of yourself. You'll get the most out of your workout without any time wasted and you'll be done before you know it. Visualize your workout. See yourself getting stronger and more confident. Get in the right mindset. Leave all worries and stress behind. Enjoy the time you're giving your body and mind by engaging in these physical challenges.

Sometimes, though, when you have had a really stressful day and you're tired and just need to get out of your head to do some stress relief, it's okay to have an easy cardio day and walk on a treadmill and not worry about anything. Or do a lightweight strength circuit including all major muscle groups for a gentle overall body workout. Always listen to your body.

But for your regular workouts, you need to include strength training at least 3 times a week. It has lots of great benefits for your health and your whole body.

The CDC recommends 2 or more days of resistance training a week in addition to cardiovascular exercise.

Besides the obvious benefits of getting stronger, maintaining muscle mass and bone strength, which are crucial to health, strength training can greatly assist you in your everyday life and functioning. "Use it or lose it" is very true for muscle mass. It's even more evident as we get older. Without strength training to maintain muscles, we start losing muscle mass in our late twenties. As our bodies produce less and less human growth hormone, we will start losing muscle every year. Even if you're not overweight, you can become "skinny fat" as you're aging and have a higher percentage of body fat than muscle mass.

Let's go over some of the most common terminology of weight training so you don't get confused.

Strength/Resistance/Weight Training:
Any exercise that causes the muscles to contract against an external resistance with the expectation of increasing strength, tone, mass, and/or endurance.

Contraction:
In working the muscles to lift the weight, they're contracted to apply force to pull or push or to maintain a position.

Isometric Contraction
Without movement. The joints remain in the

same position, like holding the plank or other poses in yoga.

Concentric:
The muscle contraction shortens the distance between the joints, as when lifting a weight.

Eccentric:
The muscle contraction lengthens the distance between joints, as when lowering a weight.

Unilateral:
Training one side of the body at a time. For example, a one-arm row will lift the weight one side with one arm, then the other side with the other arm.

Repetition/Rep:
How many times the exercise is performed. For example: doing 10 squats without stopping, you're doing 10 repetitions of squats or 10 reps.

Set:
Specific number of repetitions performed

without rest. Those 10 squats we just did will become one set of squats. Or one set of 10 repetitions.

Supersets:
Two different exercises performed back to back without rest. For example: adding 10 shoulder presses immediately after the 10 squats. They will be a super set of 10 squats and 10 shoulder presses.

Circuit:
A series of super sets. Performing one set of 10-12 repetitions of different exercises in a row with as little rest as possible. It can be repeated several times. A circuit could be a short one consisting of only about 4 exercises or a longer one with 10-12 exercises in a row, using a different muscle group in each exercise. It's great for beginners.

Periodization:
Systematic planning of training.

Compound Exercises:
Involving multiple joints and muscles

performing the exercise. For example, a squat.

Isolation Exercises:
Involving a single joint and muscle group performing the exercise. For example, a bicep curl.

Active Recovery:
Low intensity activity helping your body recover between more intense exercises or workout days.

Plateau:
When no more progress is being made. No more positive results achieved.

The best way to start is an overall body workout. Just work all muscle groups with 1 or 2 exercises. It's best to include mostly compound exercises that involve more than one joint and work more muscles at the same time. You get more done in less time. You burn more calories and you're increasing the intensity.

What do you think will burn more calories --

a dumbbell squat/curl/shoulder press move, or bicep curls alone? Especially if you're looking to lose weight, you get results much quicker with the first one, and you need to spend less time doing it.

Later on, if you decide to do more serious weight training, you can do more split routines and concentrate on different muscles.

But for a Gym Mouse, an overall body workout routine will be much more interesting and easier to follow. Do that 3 times a week and add 2 days of cardio in between. The other 2 days of the week, you can plan some outside of the gym activities with your family or just do something outside if the weather is nice. Play a sport, go on a hike, or take a class if it's not an option to go outside. If your health club has a pool, go swimming. Play tennis or basketball. Take a boxing lesson. There are different ways to stay active. Try to make your rest day an active recovery day when you don't do anything too intense, so your body can recover for your next workout, yet you are still moving.

An easy way to make the time go faster is to do your weight training as a circuit. Do one set on each machine and quickly move over to the next exercise with as little rest as possible. Do 10-12 exercises, including all major muscle groups, especially the bigger ones. Biggest muscles are in your legs, back, and chest. You want to make sure to pick exercises for those. When you're working your back and chest, you cannot help working your arms also. For now, that might be enough for them. Throw in a shoulder exercise and some core work and you'll be all set. You should concentrate on your core throughout your workout. Always check your posture. An easy way to include all those major muscles is to do the basic exercises, like squat, chest press, back row, shoulder press, plank and deadlift.

When you first start out, it's fine to use the machine equivalent of those exercises.

The next step is taking those exercises to

the cable system. They will offer some more challenges, more opportunities to work your core, your stabilizer muscles and improve your balance.

Most of the machine exercises can easily be adapted to the cable system. Ask a personal trainer to help you or, better, schedule a session to learn. It will change your workout, which will offer a new variety of exercises to make it more interesting. You'll see new and quicker results, which should help to keep you motivated to move along your fitness path to an even better, healthier you.

But your goal should be to master the free weight version of them. Free weight and body weight exercises offer more benefits and more intensity, so you can do less to see more results. They mimic real-life movements much better than machines, making them more functional and giving you results useful in your everyday life. They don't have to be complicated. Machines are bolted down and mostly make you sit with a back support, taking out the benefits of improving stabilization, balance, and core work.

You can start with some body weight moves and lighter weights until you can master form and control. Slowing the movement will make most exercises feel harder and require more effort by taking out the possibility of momentum helping you. You can make lighter weights feel heavier, giving you a more intense workout and the benefits of lifting heavier weights without putting more stress on your body if you're not ready yet. Don't be afraid of using heavier resistance when you're ready. It is beneficial for adding more muscle mass and raising your metabolism to burn more calories, even when you're resting. Most men will welcome the extra muscle on their body, but some women worry about bulking up. It's really not that easy to do for either gender. Even for men, who have more testosterone than women, it still requires a well-planned training and a nutrition and supplement program to build considerable bulk. That said, there's no reason for anyone not to improve their muscle-fat ratio, get stronger,

and have a leaner more toned and more muscular body with regular exercise.
You can also add medicine balls, exercise balls and kettle bells to your routine as you gain strength, knowledge, and interest on your journey. There are so many different ways to have fun and make the gym your playground. Don't give up! Find what you like and make that a main part of your routine.

If you can, hire a personal trainer to design an overall initial body workout for you, with the proper resistance and repetitions. Or follow the workout you received at your orientation session. That should be perfect to get you started, and when you've perfected that or you're getting a little bored with it, schedule a training session to freshen up your routine.

Keep a strong core through your exercises. That can save your lower back from getting hurt and strengthen your stomach and lower back at the same time.

A March, 2015 study by Benjamin Lee and Stuart McGill of Waterloo University showed that it's more important to develop core stiffness than to build trunk flexion fitness. Which means that planks in all variations are more beneficial and safer than sit-ups or crunches. They strengthen muscles, improve endurance, and reduce low-back pain. Sit-ups can overload the spine and lead to disc injury and chronic back pain. Exercises where you can brace your core, like a girdle, will do more for your abs and lower back than traditional crunches. Including body weight or loaded squats where you need to activate your core muscles. Push-ups and mountain climbers are also excellent examples.

There are also different classes that offer resistance training or a combination of cardio and weights. Those can be very motivating and educational. Make sure you understand the instructions and are able to follow them the right way. If something doesn't feel right, don't do it. Ask the instructor after class or ask one of the trainers to go over it with you one on one.

Weight training can be a wonderful and

rewarding experience. Don't shy away from it. Your body will thank you when you get older and can still get out of a chair or the car without help.

Think about how great a feeling it will be when you can lift something easily that gave you trouble before.

One of my clients takes great pride in how easily he can carry 40-pound bags of rock salt in the house and down to the basement for the water filter.

I'll cover the different classes in the next chapter with names and descriptions to make it easier for you to navigate through them. Try new classes, experience new things. Enjoy your discoveries!

Chapter 8:
GYM MOUSE'S GUIDE TO CLASSES

In this chapter, I'll go over the group exercise classes that your club might offer, tips on how to incorporate classes in your routine, and how to get the most out of them. They can be lots of fun! You have someone to tell you exactly what to do and watch over you to do it right. You also have others like you to share the fun with. You have music and lots of motivation. Time usually flies by and you get a great workout while having a good time.

Arrive for class on time and stay to the end. Be respectful of the instructors and your fellow members and don't interrupt the class by arriving late or leaving early.

Also, leave your phone in your locker or car. You deserve an hour of uninterrupted fun and "me" time, and the instructor and the other class participants deserve a class that's not interrupted by cell phones ringing and people talking or texting. Nothing is more distracting than a cell phone screen lighting up in a darkened yoga or cycling studio in the middle of the class. Your family should be able to reach you through the front desk in case of an unforeseen emergency. Let them know you won't have your phone on you when you're working out.

Most health clubs or gyms will offer an assortment of classes. Read the description or ask staff if you're not sure what they're all about. There might be a few different names for similar classes.

If it's a boutique studio, it will be centered around one type of exercise, like a yoga, Pilates, or cycle studio. Obviously, they're only going to have those classes or a few variations of them.

Some martial arts or boxing places might offer kickboxing or boot camp classes also.

A regular club should have cardio, strength, and combination classes. Find out the descriptions and level of the classes. Some places might offer beginner or intro classes. Sign up for those if they're available. They should be geared for beginners and new members with a slower pace and clear explanation of what the class is all about.

All classes should be doable for all levels. Instructors should provide modified versions of all exercises for beginners and less-conditioned members.

Just arrive a few minutes early to your first class and introduce yourself to the instructor and ask for help on how to modify the class. If it's a class with equipment, they will also help you with setting up what you need.

It's especially important to find out how to set up your bike for a cycle class and learn how the resistance control and brake works.

Try different classes to find out what makes you motivated and gives you a fun workout. Even try different instructors. They might have different styles, different personalities. Give them all a chance to impress you and win you over. Don't worry about not being able to do it or not being coordinated enough. You won't be the only one feeling like that. Do the best you can, pay attention to staying safe, and have fun. Who knows, you might even be a natural talent.

The dress code for classes should be the same as for the gym. Make sure your clothes are clean and light. Wear deodorant but not perfume or cologne; you may get closer to other members in a crowded class. Wear layers. Sometimes, the classrooms can be colder than the main rooms of the club if the air conditioner is blasting and the fans are on. Always have an extra shirt in case you get chilly. But wear something light also, because some smaller rooms, such as a cycle studio, can warm up quickly. Also, yoga class might have the heat on. Just be prepared for different temperatures until you figure out what works for you. Bring a workout towel and water with you to all the classes.

If you get hooked on cycling, I highly recommend that you invest in cycle shoes with cleats to clip on your bike. It makes the whole experience much better. You feel more control over the pedals and more comfortable without your feet in straps which could be too tight or get loose, allowing your feet to slide out. The cleats will also save your sneakers from extra wear and tear. For your first pair, you should go to a cycling store to get the perfect fit. Bike shoes might have European sizes, so they will be different from what you're used to. The sales people can also help you to get the right cleats to fit your gym's bikes' clips.

If you bike outside and have cycle shoes, they might fit the bikes in the gym. But if you're only going to use them in the gym, look for indoor cycle shoes. The cleats are fitted deeper in the bottom of the shoes, so they're easier to walk around with on the floor. Cleats on outside shoes stick out more, making it awkward to walk on them. Also wear shorts, capris, or narrow bottom long pants on the bike and tuck your shoelaces in. Pants and shoelaces can get caught in the pedals and wrap around them, ruining your pants, interrupting class, and making it an uncomfortable experience.

If you take Zumba or other dance classes,

you'll need Zumba or dance sneakers with a special bottom. Regular sneakers are designed to stick to the floor to prevent slipping. But when you're dancing, you need to be able to pivot. You can hurt your knees or hips if your shoes stick when they should slide. Be very careful when you first try out the class in your sport shoes. And if you plan on regularly taking them, buy the special shoes. They will enhance your experience and save you from injuries.

The club should have all the equipment and accessories you need for all the different classes, but some people like to bring their own accessories, like a mat to yoga class. If you end up taking yoga regularly, you might want to do that too.

Yoga class requires you to workout with bare feet. Keep your toenails presentable. Wear your sneakers or flip-flops to class. Don't walk through the gym barefoot. It's just not sanitary.

For most other classes, your regular sneakers will do. Some martial art classes request different shoes with thin bottoms or just bare feet.

You can wear gloves in weight training classes if you feel more comfortable with them on.

Here's a description of some of the most popular classes you might enjoy.

Water or Aqua Aerobics:
Work out in the pool, using your body weight and water resistance to get your heart rate up. Great class for beginners or the injured person doing rehabilitation and looking to avoid pounding or impact on the body.

Studio Cycling/Spinning/RPM:
Cycle class on stationary bikes with motivating music taking you through a virtual ride with sprints, races, and climbs.

Cardio Blast/Cardio Jam:
Combination of different cardio exercises, like aerobics, dance, cardio-kickboxing, high- or low-impact exercises to get your heart pumping.

Zumba, Hip-Hop, Belly Dancing, Dance:
Multi-level, choreographed dance routines
make it a high-energy, fun workout. Shaking
hips, moving abdominal muscles and
strengthening legs.

Cardio Kickboxing:
Kick and punch through a constantly moving,
fat burning class.

Step Class:
Using a step to add intensity to aerobics to
give you an overall body workout. May be
adding light dumbbells to the routine.

Boot Camp:
Military-inspired, circuit-style class improving
power, strength, and agility through a full
body workout.

Total Body Conditioning:
Cross-training for overall fitness. Mix of
cardio, step, and weights.

Sculpt, Strength, Body Pump:
Non-aerobic workout with body sculpting and
weight training in a group form. Using

dumbbells, barbells, body bars, bands, and other resistance equipment.

Yoga (various styles):
Flow through movements to increase flexibility, balance, focus, mind, and body awareness and to strengthen core and lower back.

Mat Pilates:
Improving core strength, alignment, flexibility, and promoting a healthy back.

There are special population classes offered such as:
Senior Fit or Silver Sneakers, Prenatal classes or classes designed for children or teenagers.

Also, some facilities offer a variety of Martial Arts classes. Check schedules and descriptions if you're interested.

If you still feel uncomfortable taking a class, even though you really want to, try the cycle class. It has a reputation for being a very tough class, which it is when you're ready for the intensity it offers. But it's one of the easier classes to modify. Think about it: you're on your own bike, you control your bike's resistance, and you control the speed. You can slow down when you need to; you can lower or add resistance as you see fit. Most places dim the lights for the class and everybody else will be busy with their own workout. So you can "hide in plain sight." I'm willing to bet you'll feel great after the class. Then you'll realize that classes aren't so scary; you can do other ones.

Classes can be a great way to ease into an active lifestyle, or they can be the choice of fitness activity for the rest of your life. They provide a variety of workout routines that also keep changing, so you don't get bored and keep seeing results. They will give you expert help, fun times, workout partners, and an ongoing motivation to show up.

In the next chapter, I'll go over some concerns for special conditions such as pregnancy, some chronic conditions and injuries, and different age group considerations, and how you can still have a satisfying and enjoyable workout experience in the gym.

# Chapter 9:
## SPECIAL POPULATIONS, HEALTH CONDITIONS, AND CONSIDERATIONS

There are some conditions and populations that warrant special considerations when starting or continuing an exercise program -- such as age, injuries, chronic illness and health conditions, obesity, or pregnancy.

As long as you have consulted your health practitioner and are aware of any limitations and guidelines, you should be able to lead an active life and make regular exercise a part of it.

One of my clients I worked with had MS. After months of training, she gave me a beautiful card explaining how I saved her life. She was depressed about her illness; she was smoking and felt horrible all around. Once she started training with me, she stopped smoking, used the money to buy regular training sessions, lost weight, got stronger, and her life improved on all fronts. She was happy and felt capable of managing her life and her condition.

It doesn't matter how old you are or what health problems or limitations you have, exercise can enhance the quality and the length of your life.

Do what you enjoy and what feels good! Become a healthier and better functioning Gym Mouse!

Reasonable, regular exercise can increase your energy, help maintain ideal weight, strengthen bones, muscles, joints, ligaments and tendons, lift your mood, and reduce anxiety and depression. It may even reverse or make health problems easier to manage.

It's important to always use proper technique and follow the necessary precautions. A warm up and cool down is even more important when there are special circumstances present. Use the full range of motion and address all major muscle groups.

Try all exercises without added resistance first to ensure perfect technique and test the exercises to see if they work for you and your condition. Listen to your body and don't overexert yourself. Be consistent and keep track of your progress. Be aware of proper breathing and posture. Reassess periodically to make appropriate changes.

Ensure proper intake of fluids and nutrition.

Check with your doctor to see if any of the medications you're taking can have an effect on your heart rate or blood pressure or anything else that warrants altering exercise intensity or duration.

Age concerns: seniors and juniors.

Under 14 years of age and over 65, you should get a doctor's approval and/or prescription to exercise. Even if you're in good health, it's better to have your doctor check you out. In most cases, your physician will be happy that you're planning to add an exercise regimen to your lifestyle, but there could be several reasons to modify that exercise program.

It's highly recommended that preadolescents

and teenagers participate in an hour of physical activity every day to stay healthy. It can help improve their mood, sharpen their mind, and help their skin by improving circulation and detoxification.

A cardiovascular program can help them lose or maintain weight and reduce stress and anxiety. Classes can also add a lot of fun and motivation to their regimen.

Preadolescents and adolescents need to be concerned about still growing bones and joints. They need to be avoiding competitive weightlifting, powerlifting, bodybuilding and maximal lifts until they reach physical and skeletal maturity. A carefully planned out and progressively increasing resistance training will provide benefits without injury. Ask your doctor and an informed personal trainer for advice.

Seniors needs to be concerned with weaker bones, joints, tendons, and ligaments. If there are no health problems, they should be able to follow a variety of cardio and strength programs designed for them. If you've been exercising for years, you can follow a more intense program. You just have to listen to your body and keep up with any changes in your health or strength and energy, then modify your program accordingly.

If you're starting an exercise program in your golden years, you need to follow any guidelines your doctor will give you and find a personal trainer who can help you get safely started. Mention any heart condition, chest pain, dizziness, shortness of breath, bone and joint problems, and blood pressure or cardiac medications.

Start everything gradually and listen to your body. Don't overdo it! Too much too soon will leave you exhausted, disappointed, and hurting. Slow and steady is the way to go.

Depending on your health and present shape, start with only a few minutes of walking or biking and lifting a 2-5 lbs. weight 8-10 times. Then observe how you're feeling the next day. If you're in pain or discomfort or overly tired, slow down. If you're feeling well, then gradually over a few weeks increase the time and pace of your walking and/or biking. Maybe try a different machine, such as the elliptical trainer, rowing machine, or the arm cycle. Learn to monitor your heart rate. See Chapter 6 for guidelines, or follow your physician's recommendations.

Once you can lift the weights for 2 to 3 sets of 15-20 times, increase the weight and drop back to the repetitions of 8-10 again. Ask a personal trainer to show you some age and health appropriate exercises. Also, include stretching and balance movements. Stretching should feel good and never be forced. Hold for 10-30 seconds. Some gyms have a stretching machine that assist you to get in the right position and get a better stretch. Ask a trainer to show you how to use it. It's best to take a few personal training sessions to learn the proper technique for all exercises and stretches.

Aim for a minimum of 20-30 minutes of exercise 3 to 5 times a week.

If you're injured or coming back from injury, follow your doctor's or physical therapist's recommendations. You can continue doing the exercises you learned in therapy.

Avoid taking painkillers before exercise; they can mask pain and discomfort, risking injury again by overworking still weak areas. Pain is a signal that something is wrong and it needs your attention. Don't ignore it and don't cover it up to fool you into a false sense of well-being. You can make an injury worse, and it can sideline you longer. Discuss with your doctor how to manage pain and injury while staying active through recovery and rehabilitation. Don't overdo it; too much too soon will work against you. Again, listen to your body. Also, see how you're feeling the next day. It's an important measure of how much you can handle during recovery.

Certain medications can affect your breathing, heart rate, or muscle strength. Check with your doctor to see what precautions you need to take.

Other health conditions and concerns:

Diabetes:
Physical activity can help you achieve and keep a healthy weight and keep your blood glucose levels on target. Ask your doctor's advice on how to monitor your blood sugar during and after exercise, and use snacks to prevent it from dropping too low.

High blood pressure:
An exercise program can help lower blood pressure and may help reduce or avoid medication. It can also strengthen your heart and manage your stress level, which will also be good for your blood pressure. Always check with your doctor for guidelines.

COPD, asthma, or other breathing problems: Good posture and proper breathing is a must. Physical activity will improve the muscle's' ability to get oxygen into the blood and strengthen respiratory muscles.

Arthritis:
Low-impact aerobics, strength training, range of motion exercises, and stretching can help stiff joints, build muscles, and improve endurance. Of course, when your

joints are inflamed, you need to take it easy. Short bouts of exercises may be more beneficial. Cut back on intensity if you're experiencing too much pain a couple of hours after activity.

Osteoporosis:
Good posture is a must. Avoid flexing the spine (bending forward). Exercises that gently stretch and extend your upper back will improve your posture. Work on leg muscles to improve balance and reduce the risk of falling. Strength training will work directly on your bones to slow mineral loss. Weight bearing activities like walking, dancing, low impact aerobics will also help strengthen legs and improve or maintain bone density. Swimming and water aerobics will help in rehabilitation, but will not improve bone strength because of the lack of impact or weight bearing.

Obesity:
Start slowly, increase activities gradually. As you lose weight and other health problems improve, you can add time, intensity, and new exercises to your routine.

Prenatal Fitness:

Staying active throughout your pregnancy is very important; as long as you don't have any medical conditions that would contradict exercise, there should be no reason not to continue a modified routine if you were working out regularly before your pregnancy. Even if you were not, you can definitely pick up a more active lifestyle under the care of your doctor and a personal trainer who is knowledgeable about prenatal guidelines.

One of my first clients years ago came to me after her first baby was born. She wanted to lose weight and get in shape. She did not exercise while she was pregnant, gained more than 50 pounds and had gestational diabetes, high blood pressure, and other complications. The childbirth was very hard and not a pleasant experience for her. She trained hard with me to get in shape and regained her health. She was in better shape than before the first pregnancy. Then she became pregnant again. We worked together all through her pregnancy and she was very surprised at how different this experience was. She had more energy, no complications, and a much easier time in the delivery room. She also weighed a full 100 pounds less at 9 months this time than with the previous baby.

Exercising through pregnancy can help with a healthy weight gain and increased energy; it can help to avoid health problems and complications during pregnancy and childbirth. Women who stay active during pregnancy, experience fewer common prenatal discomforts such as constipation, back pain, swollen extremities, insomnia, fatigue.

Check with your doctor for specific directions for your personal condition.

General guidelines for the pregnant exerciser:

* Be mindful of your condition. Reduce overall intensity, even if you were a regular exerciser before your pregnancy. Always listen to your body and respect any warning signs, no matter how minor they seem, and

discuss them with your doctor immediately.

* Avoid overheating. (Baby cannot sweat)

* Wear loose, comfortable clothing that facilitates heat loss. Wear a supportive bra and maternal supportive belt if needed or supportive underwear.

* Eat a pre-exercise snack and be well hydrated. Drink 6-8 ounces of water for every 15-20 minutes of activity.

* Don't exercise to exhaustion. If it's causing too much fatigue, decrease intensity or duration.

* Keep your heart rate under 140 beats per minute. Base intensity on perceived exertion.

* Modify exercises that feel awkward or uncomfortable. Focus on posture and maintain good alignment. Changes in gravity can challenge your balance and relaxed ligaments will result in looser joints.

* It's not safe lying in a supine position while exercising after the 1st trimester.

* Postnatal exercise can help to regain pre-pregnancy shape and weight, increase energy and strength, lift mood, and reduce stress and postpartum depression. It will improve self-esteem and sense of well-being.

So no matter what's going on in your life you can still make the gym part of your routine to enhance your life and get more out of it every day. It can improve your strength, your balance, and even your outlook on your life and your condition.

In the next chapter, I'll show you more of the benefits that exercising can give you, maybe some that you would never think of and some that could become your greatest motivation.

Chapter 10
BENEFITS OF EXERCISE – AND WHY
THEY MATTER

By now, you can probably see a lot of benefits of exercise. Let's see why it's a must in our modern lives.

Did you ever think about how many modern conveniences make us even less active and sedentary? We don't even have to get out of the car to bank or get a cup of coffee. We can do laundry or dishes with a push of a button. We don't have to get up to change a channel. All these convenient inventions make us less and less active every day.

Even when we should be forced to walk, we step on escalators and moving sidewalks. Our bodies need to move to stay healthy and function right. The body and the mind need the physical stress to work well. If we take that away by using all the technology to help us get more done, we need to find time to add activity back into our routine in the gym.

In my 20 years of working in the fitness industry, the biggest reason people started an exercise program was appearance. They simply wanted to look better. And that, of course, is one of the benefits. When you look better, you feel better, you have more confidence, your mood will improve, and it can give you the motivation you need to improve other areas of your life.

Besides looking better, there are a number of other health benefits. Exercise will reduce the effects of stress in all aspects of your life. It will give you a break from concentrating on work, family, and other problems.

You can take care of yourself instead of relying on others.

It can give you physical, emotional, and mental improvements. They're all connected and help each other improve in return. So one improvement can snowball into other benefits across the board.

Physical benefits include becoming stronger and having more energy and endurance to do things better, maybe even doing things you couldn't do before, making you a lot more functional in your everyday life. That again will improve your confidence and outlook on life.

All that will give you other mental and emotional improvements. As all areas of your life get better, you might even have more confidence to do more at the gym, maybe try a new class or a new equipment, which will again help you get stronger and healthier.

Activity can reverse lots of the negative effects of a sedentary lifestyle such as aches and pains, back problems, and joint stiffness, and improve your cardiovascular health, digestion and elimination, reducing constipation and improving detoxification. It can improve cholesterol, blood pressure, and other health problems. It can keep you from losing bone density and muscle mass. It will slow down the aging process inside and out, keeping you looking and feeling younger.

Exercise will help you lose weight or maintain a healthy weight more easily than just watching your diet. It will increase insulin sensitivity, preventing diabetes and obesity.

Just keep in mind that when you're doing resistance training and building some muscle, the scale weight might not change much, but you'll be losing inches. Muscle is denser than fat, takes up less room, but weighs more. So you'll look better, leaner, and more toned. Don't worry about the number on the scale. If you look great, you lost inches where you needed to, you have more muscle, you're stronger and healthier, and you're on the right track.

Being active can also help fix your circadian rhythm, allowing you to sleep better so you recover faster from workouts or other physical or mental stress and have more energy to do new things you're now capable of doing.

It will strengthen the immune system to prevent illness or recover faster from being sick, and it will make us physically more resilient to injury and allow us to recover faster from any injury.

Regular physical activity will also improve mood, reduce anxiety, and depression.

So, you see that exercise will help a lot of areas of your life to get better. Keep in mind, though, that too much exercise too soon or too intense when you're not ready can be harmful.

If you're under extreme stress or having a lot of health or emotional problems, you might have to start your workout program with a gentle routine first to get your body restored enough to have enough energy to increase the intensity and duration of your workouts. Train, don't drain. These movements should be gentle, slow paced, and simple so that you can concentrate on breathing and healing and not on technique and form just yet. They should include some slow-paced walking, stretching, and gentle yoga moves. Tai Chi or Qigong are also very useful.

Once your stress load improves, gradually increase the duration and intensity of your routines. You should feel better overall. Your mood should improve and you should feel more capable of handling stress. Your energy and mental functions improve, and blood pressure and heart rate should move toward optimal. Body weight can improve and sleep will become better quality, making you more rested. Talk to a personal trainer who understands the effects of stress and the body's reaction to it so they can help you with a plan to get started.

Also, remember that the benefits of regular physical activity will be lasting as long as you're paying attention to the other components needed for good health, such as eating right, drinking water, getting enough sleep, and taking time to relax and enjoy life. We will look at how to put them all together next.

Look for more details in my other books coming out soon about easy-to-follow workout programs, healthy eating and nutrition, and stress relief.

Chapter 11:
MAKING IT HAPPEN - HOW TO BECOME
A HEALTHY GYM MOUSE

So, my dear Gym Mouse friend, by now, you know the mechanics. How to join the gym, how to get started, what to do. You know you need to do it. It doesn't look as scary as it did before you started reading. It all sounds good on paper and in your head.

Let's put all this information together and actually make it happen. It is time to do it!

Don't let negative people talk you out of your decision. They're usually just as afraid to start as you were. Turn it around on them and invite them to go with you. Help each other get started. Tell them to go with you as a guest and see how easy it is to take the first step. Turn them into a positive exercise partner. And if they still resist, just show them you can still do it and don't let them hold you back.

Start with small changes, but do them every day. Make a contract with yourself that you'll stay active every day, even if you're just going for a walk or doing 10 minutes of exercises in front of your TV. Do at least 30 minutes of activity each day. Do more if you're sitting most of the day.

Look at your schedule and put your gym time on it. Schedule it like an appointment and only cancel if it's absolutely necessary. Set attainable, reasonable goals. If you think you can get to the gym twice a week, then start with that. Create a habit. Once the 2 days per week become a routine and easily doable, add another one. You might even start enjoying it and have fun.
The best time to exercise is in the morning. It's easier to stick with it if that's the first thing on your agenda. All you have to do is get up early enough to get there. There would be less distraction than later in the day. You'll also feel better and more energetic all day, plus you've already started your day with a great accomplishment. That should give your confidence and mood a wonderful boost.

It should also make it somewhat easier to make healthier meal choices. You already got up early and worked hard to get and stay healthier. Why ruin this by eating lousy junk food?

The gym is also calmer in the morning. Less socializing, more getting on with business, because everyone has to go to work. There's more of a chance to get on the equipment you'd like to use.

You'll also get to know the crowd in the morning. Most of them will be there every day at the same time Monday through Friday. You'll make friends for sure and may even find a workout partner. You'll feel a sense of belonging when you're part of the group every day. Then you'll want to show up so you don't miss them and they don't miss you. Another reason to keep going.

If you're planning to go after work, the best way to do it is bringing your gym bag with you, so you can go straight there. No obstacles arise, as they could if you have to stop home and being home gets the best of you and deters you from going out again.

Even if you feel like you don't want to go, make a deal with yourself that you'll exercise for 15 minutes in the gym. Chances are that once you're there and get started, you'll do more. And if you don't, you accomplished what you set out do.

Of course, if you cannot do it in the early morning or after work, any time will do. I went through the pros and cons of the different times of day in Chapter 2.

Try out different times when you're available and see what time feels the best. Some people like the busy, keep moving, happening nighttime. It gives them more energy. Some people are more motivated in the morning. Do what works for you.

For a change of pace, go at different times occasionally, maybe when you're on vacation, Try new classes, new instructors. Meet new people. You might find something else you like.

Variety will keep you going and make your fitness experience more interesting. It will keep you from boredom and from overuse injuries. Also, you'll see quicker results the more variety you include in your routine.

Treat the gym as a playground. Don't make it a chore. It should be a source of joy and stress relief. Find a way to make it fun! Take classes, use the personal trainers!

Leave your phone and gadgets in your locker or car and get away from everything, body and mind. Think only of yourself and the good you're doing for your health and well-being.

Step out of your box a little and challenge yourself. You'll feel great after accomplishing new goals and seeing new results. Concentrate on positive changes, no matter how small they are.

More energy, better sleep, less anxiety, and easier stress management are all steps in the right direction. Weight loss and body composition changes will follow if you're consistent. You didn't get where you are overnight, so you cannot fix everything overnight.

Start with what you can do and enjoy. Don't give up! Gradually increase intensity, duration, and frequency.

Alternate hard with easy or active rest days. Or alternate cardio and strength days. Try it out or ask a personal trainer to help find the best routine for you.

Let your body recover between workouts. You'll be sore and little stiff after using muscles that were neglected for a while. It's okay, it's a good thing. It's a sign that you reached an intensity to challenge your body to adapt and make changes. It will be somewhat uncomfortable, but should not be debilitating. If it's that bad, you need to cut back and start slower.

When you're sore, the best thing you can do is keep moving. Some gentle exercises, stretches, or light cardio workout will make you feel better. Too much rest will make you stiffer, and once you increase intensity again, you'll be just as sore.

Going in the sauna for a short while or sitting in a hot tub should loosen you up also. So would getting a nice massage.
Expect to be sore here and there when you introduce a new form of exercise or increase the intensity, but it should be more bearable and you should recover faster the fitter you get.

Keep properly hydrated and fueled for your exercise sessions. Make changes in your nutrition choices. Part of a healthy lifestyle besides exercise is healthy eating, drinking enough water, getting enough sleep, and managing stress. Implement the 80/20 rule. Take control of the 80% of your life that you can control and make the best and healthiest choices. Then that 80% will absorb the 20% you cannot control, such as the stress from unforeseen events, and you'll be the healthiest Gym Mouse you can be.

Keep in mind that working out doesn't give you a free pass to eat anything and everything. You cannot work out a bad diet!

Unfortunately, it takes much longer to burn the calories than to consume them. Most people learn the hard way and gain weight after joining the gym. So watch the portions! Drink plenty of filtered water all day long. It will give you more energy and help you lose or maintain your weight.

Eat plenty of protein to help build muscle and keep you satisfied. Eat carbs for energy and recovery, but choose vegetables and fruits over starches and sweets. Carbs will spike your blood sugar, which will increase insulin in your blood. It's almost impossible to burn fat in the presence of a lot of insulin. Learn to keep blood sugar steady by not eating carbohydrates by themselves. The best time to consume a carbohydrate-rich meal is right after exercise. Don't forget fat! You need it to control your hormones, which have a lot to do with your weight. They also add to your satiety, making you fuller and with less cravings. Choose butter from grass-fed cows, coconut oil, and cold-pressed olive oil.

All these aspects of your lifestyle work

together and support each other or destroy each other. Fixing your diet will give you more energy and fuel to exercise, so it will improve, which will make for better stress management and sleep.

A healthier diet will lead to fewer blood sugar fluctuations, which will result in better sleep quality. That, again, will give you more energy to exercise and less craving to mess up your diet, because lack of sleep will make your body crave more sugar for quick energy and make healthier nutrition choices much harder.

Don't forget that stress is cumulative. It's not just your financial concerns or bad relationships or other problems in your life. Eating the wrong diet, not getting enough sleep, not enough exercise, or too much exercise all add to your stress level. As far as your body is concerned, there's no difference. You need to work on all areas for a balanced and less stressful life.

Less stress, more sleep, better nutrition, and more exercise will result in better health and a healthier weight. Try meditation, yoga, and other stress management techniques to work on other areas.

Don't overdo it! Listen to your body! Too much too soon can lead to injury and burnout. You might find yourself falling in love with your new lifestyle and actually enjoying exercise. It's fine to go from Gym Mouse to Gym Rat, but make sure you don't become obsessed and addicted to working out. Overtraining can be very stressful on your body and can hinder results. It can reverse the positive effects of exercising. Find the balance between activity and recovery and adequate rest.

Look for more details in my next book *on nutrition, exercise, and stress management.*

Now you have all the tools on how to get started and what to do.

It's time to find your WHY. The real reasons to join the gym and keep going. How do you motivate yourself to keep moving if you don't find health and fitness alone motivating enough on their own? It's time to find your end game: your dream.

Chapter 12:
FINDING YOUR WHY – THE REAL
REASONS TO JOIN THE GYM

Congratulations! You have accomplished
one big step. You read through my book to
learn how to get started and what to do in
the gym. That means you're interested in
making changes for the better in your life. It's
exciting, it's a new beginning. Embrace it
and enjoy every step and every minute of it.

Carl Bard wrote, "Though no one can go
back and make a brand new start, anyone
can start from now and make a brand new
ending."

Think about these words for a minute.

Think about where you want to be in a year,
in 10 years, in 20 years. How much can your
life improve or not deteriorate if you make
changes now? How do you want others to
remember you? As a strong, healthy person
who accomplished everything you set out to
do? Or someone who was weak and sick

and just barely made it through life or watched a lot of it from the sidelines?

You might think exercise cannot possibly make such a big difference. Can it really be life changing?

I've seen thousands of people come through the door over the years I've been working in the gym. I've also seen thousands quit and leave. I've also seen thousands return. It didn't matter if they enjoyed their time exercising regularly or not, they all agreed that it made a difference in their lives. They all felt better, stronger, happier, and had more energy for everything else.

Find your dream! Find your why!

Maybe you always wanted to run a 5K race or even a marathon. Maybe you wanted to climb a mountain, rollerblade with your friends, or bench press some serious weights. Or maybe you dreamed about some other fitness goals that eluded you because you were too scared to go to the gym and used every excuse to avoid it.

Deep down, you might really want to be a gym rat, but just didn't believe you can be one.

Maybe you couldn't care less about any fitness goals, just want to be healthy and be able to function every day without difficulty. But that might not be enough to motivate you to keep going every day, especially if you're fairly healthy right now and don't really like to exercise.

Don't wait until a flight of stairs will make you breathless or you can't carry a bag of groceries into the house. It's much easier to start before you get to that point, but not impossible.

Just think about how great it will be not to have to rely on other people's help for the longest possible time even in your later years. And how cool it will be to impress your grandchildren with your fitness!

It's never too late to move. It doesn't matter how slowly; it will still be faster than not moving at all.

Just the other day in the grocery store, I packed my own bag. I like to put as much in each bag as I can. The girl, who probably was half my age, couldn't lift my bag into my shopping cart with 2 hands. Not cool for her. I had no problem doing it.

Lots of people find improving appearance more motivating than anything else. If that's how you feel, great! Use that to push you to start moving.

You can concentrate on some immediate goals, like an event. A reunion or a wedding you want to look great for, a birthday or anniversary or other occasion where you have to face people whose opinions you value. Those will give you a temporary motivation, and it's wonderful. It's good to have a date and specific goal. By the time you get in shape for those events, you should have realized all the other benefits and established a routine you can easily maintain until the next goal you find.

How about finding a bigger why, a bigger dream that would give you the push to get to the gym when you don't feel like it?

I have a client who came back to train with me after a 2-year absence. She's 61 years old and has a small granddaughter whom she adores. Her greatest motivation is to be there for the baby as she grows up and to be able to play with her, take care of her, and participate in her life. After only 4 weeks of training, she was very excited to tell me that now she can play with her on the floor and she can get up by herself. And an even bigger accomplishment, she can get out of the beanbag chair now, which was impossible before. These results will keep her going.

How about being a role model for your children? All parents want the best for their children. They want them to have a better and more fulfilling life than they had. So you must want excellent health for them. Show them the example. Show them that it's possible to include exercise even in a busy life. Show them that health is important and show them that they're important enough for you to take care of your own health, so you can be there for a long time healthy and strong to take care of them and support them. Show them how to take responsibility for their bodies and lives. Teach them good practices and habits. It will make it easier for them to keep it up for the rest of their lives if that's what they learn from the beginning, and they will do the same for their children.

How about just a goal of happiness? Having a reason to get out of bed in the morning. Regular physical activity has been proven to help depression. If you suffering from that, consider exercise as a part of your recovery process.

How about stress relief? The gym is a great place to get away from every day stress and clear your head. Take a class or train with your personal trainer to give your mind a break from everything else. Just think about your body and enjoying the physical energy and relief. Just make sure you listen to your body. Some days, when stress is too much in your life, don't add to it with too much or too intense exercise. On those days, you'll need some form of activity that's gentler.

Take a yoga or a stretching class or a dance class and just enjoy the music and fun. Don't worry about the perfect steps or just take a walk and let your mind relax. Let your trainer know what's going on so they can help you recover with the appropriate exercises.

How about being more productive and successful at work? When you're in shape and have more energy and a better state of mind, you'll make a better impression on people, get more done, and be able to deal with people and anything coming your way.

Maybe you will even gain the confidence to go out and get the job you really want?

So there are several reasons that being active can enhance your life. Think about your end game. Think about what you want for yourself and how being stronger can help you reach those goals. Then it will be easier to take the first step toward the new you.

Get started now with your new beginning and change your ending.

Send me an email and tell me your why at agi@healthbalanced.com. Maybe, together, we can help other Gym Mouse friends to find their dreams.

# BEGINNER WORKOUT FOR THE GYM MOUSE

Ask your medical professional's advice before starting this or any other exercise program.


CARDIO INTERVAL WORKOUT - Do this twice a week:

On a stationary bike, rowing machine, or elliptical machine:

1. Warm up 3-5 minutes at a moderate pace.

Work 30 seconds as hard as you can.  (Add resistance and/or go faster)
Rest 45-60 seconds.  (Slow down to an easy pace to recover)
Repeat 4 times.

Rest 1 minute.  (Easy pace)

Repeat above workout 1-2 times.

Cool down 3-5 minutes at a moderate to slow pace.

As you get stronger, switch to:

2.  Warm up 3-5 minutes at a moderate pace.

Work 30 seconds as hard as you can.
Rest 30 seconds. (Easy pace to recover)
Repeat 4 times

Rest 1 minute (easy pace)

Repeat above workout 3-4 times.

Cool down 3-5 minutes. (Easy pace)

RESISTANCE TRAINING - do this 3 times a week. (Alternate with cardio workout)

Pick the weights so you can complete the 12 repetitions with good form, yet it's somewhat challenging. Start with 1 set and work it up to 3 sets. Rest as needed between exercises. Ask a trainer for machine set up and to check your form.

8-10 minute warm up on any cardio equipment at slow to moderate pace.

2-3 sets of:

12 repetitions on the Seated Row Machine alternated with
12 repetitions of Body Weight Squats (lower hips toward floor as low as you can go while keeping your heels on the floor, then "push the floor away" with feet as you're coming back up, try to go lower than thighs parallel to the floor)

12 reps on the Chest Press Machine (exhale as you lift, inhale as you lower weight) alternated with 12 reps each leg of Side Leg Lifts (stand on one leg and slowly raise and lower the other leg to the side. Try not to touch your foot to the ground between repetitions.)

12 reps Straight Mountain Climbers (on hands and feet, aim your left knee toward your left elbow as you pull them into your chest. Alternate legs)

12 reps Cross Body Mountain Climbers (aim left knee to right elbow then switch sides)

12 reps Lying Down Hip-lifts. (Lie on your back with knees bent and feet on the floor close to your buttocks. Lift hips toward ceiling as you squeeze your gluteus muscles, and then slowly lower.)

5 minutes on the Rowing Machine at a moderate pace to loosen muscles and cool down.

## ABOUT THE AUTHOR:

## Agi Kadar

Agi was born in Budapest, Hungary. She participated in several sports from a young age, starting with swimming, gymnastics, and basketball. Then, as a teenager, she competed in fencing until she relocated to New York at the age of 20.

Starting a new life, she was too busy to participate in formal sports, so she started running outside. Eventually, that led to numerous road races from 5K races to full 26.2-mile marathons. She finished 14 marathons: 10 in New York City, 3 in Budapest and 1 in Boston. Agi also helped a number of disabled athletes finish the New York City Marathon as a guide.

Agi Kadar has been in the fitness industry for over 20 years, working in the same gym for the last 16.

She has a degree in Exercise Science, Personal Trainer and Corrective Exercise

Specialist Certifications from NASM (National Academy of Sports Medicine), and RPM (cycle instructor) Certification from Les Mills. She is a Metabolic Typing Advisor, Holistic Lifestyle Coach, Functional Nutrition Practitioner, and has Lower Body Solution and Kickboxing Certificates.

She takes classes constantly and reads to keep up with the latest information so she can offer the best possible advice to her clients.

She spends a lot of time training clients one on one or in group settings and listens to their concerns, fears, and helps them achieve their goals to become successful, healthy adults.

She always had a heart to help those who were scared and didn't think they could be successful in a fitness facility. Over the years, she led classes and small training groups to make it easier for those who didn't want to do it alone.

Agi's greatest reward is to see each one's

transformation from a scared little Gym Mouse to a confident and proud member of the gym: achieving and exceeding their goals and greatly improving their lives along the way.

She is very excited to be able to combine her passions: training, helping people become healthier and happier, and writing about it.

Agi Kadar lives, works, trains and writes in Carmel, New York.

Please look for more information on Agi's website: www.areyouagymmouse.com and in her next books focusing on Nutrition, Training Routines, and Stress Management.

Agi is always open for questions and feedback at agi@healthbalanced.com.

Thank you for purchasing my book! Please help my next books to be even better by leaving your feedback with a helpful review on Amazon.

45427494R00086

Made in the USA
Middletown, DE
03 July 2017